The

LITTLE BOOK OF

YOGA

Haf.

X, Pat.

THE LITTLE BOOK OF YOGA

An Hachette UK Company
www.hachette.co.uk

Summersdale Publishers Ltd
Part of Octopus Publishing Group Limited
Carmelite House
50 Victoria Embankment
LONDON
EC4Y 0DZ
UK

www.summersdale.com

Printed and bound in Malta

ISBN: 978-1-78685-280-9

Substantial discounts on bulk quantities of Summersdale books are available to corporations, professional associations and other organisations. For details contact general enquiries: telephone: +44 (0) 1243 771107 or email: enquiries@summersdale.com.

The

LITTLE BOOK OF

YOGA

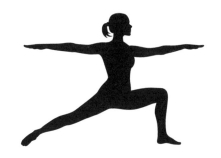

Eleanor Hall

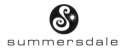

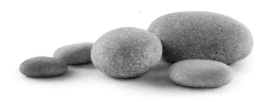

INTRODUCTION

AT THE CENTRE OF YOGA IS YOU.

Yoga helps to build harmony between your body and mind, taking you on a journey to a stronger, calmer, healthier and happier you. By picking up this book you have taken the first step on your yoga path.

With this little book I hope to encourage some of you to start a regular yoga practice and enjoy all the wonderful benefits it has to offer.

YOU CANNOT DO YOGA.
YOGA IS YOUR NATURAL
STATE. WHAT YOU CAN
DO ARE YOGA EXERCISES,
WHICH MAY REVEAL TO YOU
WHERE YOU ARE RESISTING
YOUR NATURAL STATE.

SHARON GANNON

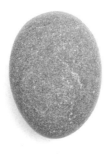

GETTING
STARTED

THE MOST IMPORTANT PIECES OF EQUIPMENT YOU NEED FOR DOING YOGA ARE YOUR BODY AND YOUR MIND.

RODNEY YEE

PREPARING FOR YOUR PRACTICE

Wear comfortable, stretchy – but not loose – clothes. It's best to practise in bare feet and on a non-slip yoga mat.

Roll out your yoga mat in a calm, warm and quiet space, which has enough room for you to stretch out your arms to each side.

Yoga is best practised before a meal as it is better if you have an empty stomach. You should also ensure you are fully hydrated.

Try to designate time for your practice each week. You can practise as little or as often as you want, however the body does respond well to a regular practice – just 10 minutes a day can be as beneficial as an hour's class a week.

Special conditions

Traditionally it has been suggested that inverted postures, strong twists and back bends be avoided during menstruation, but the best advice is to practise what suits you.

Women who are pregnant should consult a doctor before beginning any practice and starting a new practice is not advised during your first trimester.

If you are concerned for any reason or suffer from a particular health condition or injury please consult a doctor before starting.

It is important to remember yoga is not a competition, it is about finding a connection with your body and your mind – not about being more flexible than the person on the next mat, or being able to tie yourself into a knot. Pace yourself and observe your body at all times, responding to how you feel.

Everybody is different – postures that come easily to others may be difficult for you and vice versa. Don't become disheartened if a pose doesn't come naturally to you or feels almost impossible to begin with.

Breathing is vital to achieving a successful yoga practice, so make sure you follow the breath cues within each pose to inhale and exhale, and then aim to hold each posture for five deep breaths. Be sure to work with your body, moving slowly and steadily into each posture, stopping when you feel you have comfortably reached your full potential.

Most importantly... enjoy!

BREATHING

Pranayama

The importance of breathing in yoga is often overlooked: breath is our life force and energy. The Sanskrit word *prana* represents all three and the practice of pranayama is where breath is controlled to increase energy, focus and consciousness.

Within our practice the breath helps us to calm the mind, build focus and deepen our postures. We use our inhale to lift, lengthen and open the body, and our exhale to release, soften and ground us.

It is important to stay focused to your breath throughout your practice, feeling the connection of each movement with your breath. The traditional Sun Salutation practice (see page 38) is often used at the start of a practice to warm up the body, start the body flowing and help that connection of your movements with your breath.

A good way to start any yoga session is with a restorative pose such as Corpse Pose (see page 19) or Child's Pose (see page 25). Take a moment here to calm the mind and body and start bringing your focus to your breath. Start to feel the breath coming in and out of your body; breathing through your nose, notice the cold air on the inhale and the warm air on the exhale. Try to keep your attention on your breath and the feelings within your body; try to detach from any other thoughts and bring yourself to this moment on your mat.

You can then start to try to lengthen your breath, trying to count your inhale in for the count of five and exhale to the count of eight. By lengthening our exhale we help to detoxify the body, still the mind and relieve stress.

Once you feel comfortable and connected here start to move into a gentle warm up (see page 32), followed by Sun Salutations and a mixture of postures from this book. Always ensure you finish any practice with a Corpse Pose.

WHEN THE BREATH WANDERS,
THE MIND IS UNSTEADY, BUT
WHEN THE BREATH IS STILL,
SO IS THE MIND STILL.

YOGA PRADIPIKA

CORPSE POSE

Savasana

Corpse Pose is the well-known relaxation that we take at the end of any yoga practice. In some practices it is also used at the start of the class to tune into your body and breath, helping to calm your mind in preparation for your practice.

While this is a relaxation pose it can be surprisingly difficult to begin with, as we struggle to switch off our busy minds – not allowing ourselves to enjoy the peace and quietness within our bodies – and we can feel restless and even vulnerable with our eyes closed and in the openness of the pose.

However, once you can relax and surrender to this pose it creates a feeling of deep relaxation and inner peace, allowing you to release tension and stresses in the body and mind, as well as absorbing all the benefits of your practice.

Step by step

1. Lying with your back and legs flat to your mat, place your arms at your sides with your palms facing up. Close your eyes and bring your attention to your breath, allowing deep breaths in and out of your nose. Then start to bring your attention to each area of your body, allowing your whole body to relax back into the mat.

2. Widen your legs flat on your mat, allow them to relax and let your feet roll out to the sides. Lift your buttocks slightly, lengthening through your lower back and bringing your sacrum and spine flat to the mat. Tuck your chin in to lengthen the back of your neck and feel your neck as an extension of your spine.

3. Soften your shoulders so they almost melt into the floor. Allow your arms and hands to be heavy and relaxed, sinking into the mat.

4. Release any tension in your forehead and soften the eyebrows and skin around your eyes, allowing your

eyes to feel as though they're sinking back in their sockets. Unclench your teeth, relax your jaw and detach your tongue from the roof of your mouth.

5. Ensure there is no tension and allow the mat to take the weight of your whole body. Bring your attention back to your breath, feel the inhale coming fully into the body, flowing down to your fingers and toes, and as you exhale feel any lasting tension or stresses releasing with your breath.

6. Try to detach yourself from any thoughts, only allowing thoughts to pass through your mind, and keep bringing your attention back to your breath. Melt into your mat and feel softness across your whole body.

7. Stay here for at least five minutes for every 60 minutes of practice.

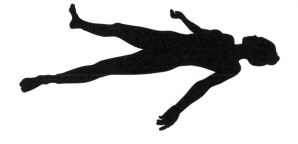

IN THE MIDST OF MOVEMENT AND CHAOS, KEEP STILLNESS INSIDE OF YOU.

DEEPAK CHOPRA

CHILD'S POSE

Bālāsana

**Child's Pose is a wonderful restorative
pose to help elongate your spine, soothe
back pain and open your hips. Throughout
your practice it can be used as a rest pose
between the more challenging postures.**

Step by step

1. Kneel on your mat. Bring your big toes together, sit back onto your heels and separate your knees as wide as your hips.

2. Bend at the waist and lie down onto your legs, resting your torso on your thighs and your forehead on the mat. Lay your arms alongside your body with your palms facing up. Widen your shoulder blades across your back and lengthen your neck. Feel your tailbone drawing back towards your heels.

3. Alternatively, you can stretch your arms out in front of you, palms down. Keep your shoulders back from your ears and lengthen your neck and spine forwards.

4. As a resting pose you can hold here for 30 seconds or a few minutes. To come out of this pose, bring your hands underneath your shoulders and slowly roll the spine up to bring you sitting back onto your heels.

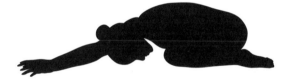

ALTERNATE NOSTRIL BREATHING

Nadi Shodhana

As well as keeping the connection to your breath throughout your practice there are also some specific breathing exercises you can do to help your body and mind in different ways. Alternate nostril breathing balances the left and right sides of our brain and is therefore wonderful for relieving tension and stress, as well as promoting a feeling of balance in the body. It is also great for promoting good sleep. This exercise can be done before or after your practice.

Step by step

1. Sitting in a comfortable position on your mat, ensure your spine is straight, the crown of your head reaching upwards.

2. Rest your left hand on your knee and lift your right hand, placing your first two fingers onto your third eye, which is the area at the top of your nose between your eyebrows. Place your thumb gently on your right nostril and your third finger on your left nostril.

3. Close your eyes, lift your spine and ground your sitting bones into the floor. Close off your left nostril with your finger and exhale completely from your right.

4. Inhale through your right nostril to the count of five, close the right nostril with your thumb and release the left, exhale through your left nostril to the count of five. Inhale through your left nostril to the count of five, close your left side and release your thumb to exhale through your right side to the count of five.

This is one round. Try to complete five rounds and then release your hand back to your knee to take a few normal breaths.

5. Try to do three sections of five rounds, resting between each. Alternatively try to increase the counts by taking section two as an inhale for five counts and exhale for ten counts, then for your third section add breath retention by holding your breath for five counts after each inhale and then continuing.

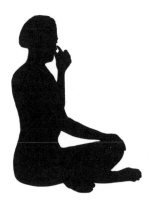

BREATHING IS ONE OF THE GREATEST SECRETS OF YOGA – IF YOU PRACTISE, IT WILL OBTAIN EMOTIONAL POWERS BEYOND YOUR IMAGINATION.

BIJA BENNETT

WARM-UP EXERCISES

Start any practice with a warm up to prepare your whole body. This will help you to deepen and lengthen the hold of each posture, prevent injury and increase fluidity in your body. It will also help oxygen and energy to circulate through your body.

Gently lengthen or rotate each of your joints and muscles starting with your spine. A great way to do this is with the Cat and Cow poses: see page 36–37 for how to enter these postures.

Other great warm-up stretches include:

Neck rolls – Drop your chin towards your chest, roll your head to the right and bring your right ear towards your right shoulder. Continue to roll your head back and then round to the left to bring your left ear to your left shoulder. Do this a couple of times and then do the same in the other direction.

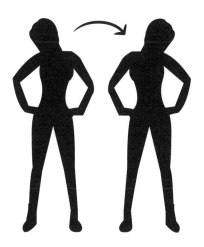

Shoulder rolls - Lift your shoulders and roll them down your back, then round to the front and back up. Do this a couple of times and then round to the front first.

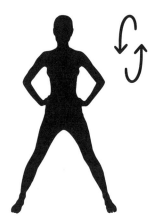

Seated side stretches - Sitting cross-legged, lift your arms above your head. Bring your left hand to the mat, stretching your right arm over your head, reaching your fingers to the left. Hold for a few deep breaths and repeat on the other side.

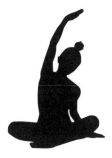

Extension and flexing of wrists and ankles – Hold your arms out in front of you, turn your fingers up to the sky and then down towards the floor. Repeat five times. Sit with your legs out in front of you, flex your toes towards your face and then point them down to the floor. Repeat five times.

Try to do each of these exercises before starting your practice.

CAT AND COW POSE

Kneel down on your mat then go on to all fours, with your knees directly underneath your hips and your shoulders stacked above your wrists.

Inhale as you drop your navel down, lifting your tailbone to curve your spine downwards. Lift your head, rolling your shoulders back down your back to open across your chest. Keep your arms straight and take your gaze up to the sky. This is Cow Pose.

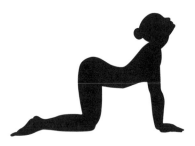

On your exhalation, round your back to lift the spine upwards, widening across the shoulder blades and engaging your abdominal muscles to draw your navel back towards your spine. Ensure that you are rolling through the whole spine as you round your back upwards – it can be easy to arch the upper back, so ensure you are pushing through the lower back as well. Drop your head towards the floor and press the tops of your feet and the palms of your hands into your mat. This is Cat Pose.

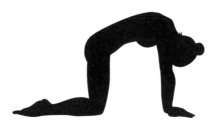

Repeat a couple of rounds moving as fluidly and gently as possible from Cow to Cat to warm up the back, moving the spine gently with each inhalation and exhalation.

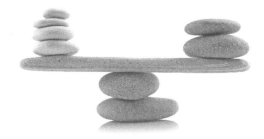

SUN
SALUTATIONS

Sun Salutations are a well-known traditional part of many yoga practices. They are a wonderful way to start your yoga practice as they limber up and awaken your whole body, deepen your breathing and improve breath control. As the name would suggest, Sun Salutations are a great way to start the day as you greet the sun and wake up your body and mind.

With regular practice this sequence of movements will become more graceful and flowing. Don't forget to try to keep each movement connected to an inhale or exhale – this also will become easier with regular practice. Try to complete three to five rounds at the beginning of each practice, or on their own as the perfect mini practice to start your day.

Following are the postures you will need to learn to complete your Sun Salutations.

MOUNTAIN POSE

Tadasana

While this may look like you're simply standing up straight, this surprisingly strong pose is an important one which you can start with and return to in your practice. It will help you to find your space on the mat, ground you to the earth and connect you back to your breath.

Step by step

1. Stand at the top of your mat with your heels together. Place your arms down by your sides with your palms facing in. Fingers should be engaged as they lengthen towards the mat.

2. Close your eyes and take a moment to bring your attention to each area of your body. Start by lifting your toes, spreading them wide apart and then lowering them back onto the mat, becoming aware of each toe connected to the mat. Then notice the balls of your feet and the soles of your feet as you spread your weight evenly over each foot.

3. Straighten your legs, bringing your knees directly over your ankles and your hips directly over your knees. Engage your thighs, lifting your kneecaps and strengthening your legs. Support this movement by tucking your tailbone under and engaging your core (abdominal muscles).

4. Now take your attention to your spine, feel yourself lifting and lengthening as you draw the crown of your head towards the sky. Open your chest as you roll your shoulders back, lengthening your arms at your sides.

5. Draw your chin slightly down to lengthen the back of your neck. Stand tall and connect to your breathing.

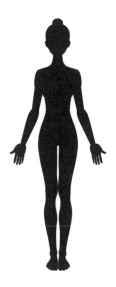

DEEP FORWARD FOLD POSE

Uttanasana

This deep fold gives an intense stretch to your hamstrings and spine, and allows a softening in your neck and shoulders, increasing the blood flow to your brain, helping you to calm your mind and feel restored and refreshed.

Step by step

1. Stand in Mountain Pose (see page 40) at the top of your mat. Inhale as you lift your arms above your head, joining your palms together. Allow your gaze to follow your arms as they lift, watching your palms as they join.

2. Tuck your tailbone under and engage your lower belly. Exhale as you fold forwards, hinging from the hips. Keep drawing your navel back towards your spine and make your spine long as you fold towards the knees.

3. Place your hands on the floor either side of your feet. If you can't reach your hands to the floor, bend your knees a little. Press your palms to the floor, spreading your fingers and engaging with your mat.

4. Draw your shoulders back, lengthening your neck, and tuck your chin slightly under. Allow gravity to draw the crown of your head closer to the mat.

5. Take five deep breaths. If your legs are bent, allow them to gently straighten with each exhale.

6. Inhale as you lift up bringing your palms back together above your head. Exhale as you lower your hands to come into Mountain Pose.

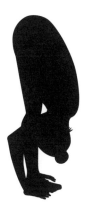

DOWNWARD-FACING DOG POSE

Adho Mukha Śvānāsana

As one of the most widely recognised yoga poses, Downward-Facing Dog is used in the traditional Sun Salutation sequence as well as being a wonderful yoga pose on its own for an all over energising stretch.

Step by step

1. Come onto your mat on your hands and knees, with your knees directly below your hips and your hands slightly above your shoulders. Spread your fingers, and connect your palms and each fingertip with the mat.

2. Tuck your toes under and lift your knees away from the mat, start to lengthen and lift your tailbone away from your pelvis, lifting your sitting bones towards the ceiling.

3. Push your thighs back, feel your chest softening back towards your knees and draw your heels towards the floor. Straighten your legs but be careful not to lock your knees.

4. Draw your shoulders away from your ears, widening your shoulder blades and drawing them back towards your tailbone. Feel your spine lengthen and straighten, keeping your back flat. Your head should be between your upper arms, with your gaze towards your navel.

5. Hold pose for five deep breaths, then bend your knees back down to the mat and draw your sitting bones back towards your heels, coming into Child's Pose.

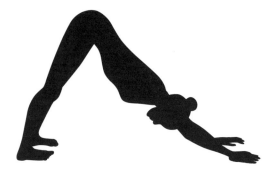

UPWARD-FACING DOG POSE

Ūrdhva Mukha Śvānāsana

Upward-Facing Dog is a rejuvenating stretch that works your whole spine, opens your chest, tones your belly and strengthens your arms and wrists.

Step by step

1. Lie flat, with your forehead resting on the mat, and the tops of your feet flat to the mat and hip width apart.

2. Place your hands to the sides of your body, palms flat to the mat, fingers pointing forwards with your fingertips in line with your shoulders. Tuck your toes under and inhale as you press your hands into the mat and lift your body away from the floor. Start to pull your hips forwards as you roll over your toes so the tops of your feet are flat to the mat.

3. Straighten your arms and lift your chest forwards: feel like you're pulling your chest through your arms. Make sure your legs are straight and engaged, keeping the thighs and knees lifted off the mat. The weight of your body should be spread evenly over your hands and feet.

4. Roll your shoulders back and down, tilt your head back slightly and take your gaze up.

5. Soften your shoulders, pulling them down your back, opening across the chest. Tuck your chin in towards your throat, keeping the neck long.

6. Hold for five deep breaths, expanding your chest and lengthening your spine with each breath. To release, bend your knees to the mat and exhale as you slowly lower all the way down to the mat.

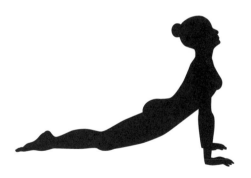

FOUR-LIMBED STAFF POSE

Chaturanga Dandasana

Four-Limbed Staff Pose is great for full body strengthening. As the weight of your body rests on your hands and feet, you are working your arms, wrists, shoulders and core.

Step by step

1. Start on your mat in a plank position, with your shoulders stacked above your wrists, fingers pointing forwards, feet hip distance apart. Push your heels back, ensuring your shoulders and wrists are still stacked.

2. Engage your abdominal muscles and slowly start to move the shoulders forwards to your fingertips as you bend into your elbows. Before lowering, turn your inner elbows to face into each other to keep them hugged into the body and avoid them pushing outwards.

3. Keep slowly lowering until your elbows are bent at right angles and the tops of your arms are in line with your chest. Ensure your whole body is straight, avoid lifting your buttocks and keep your neck in line with your spine, with your gaze lowered.

4. Hold for five deep breaths. Exhale as you slowly lower all the way down to the mat.

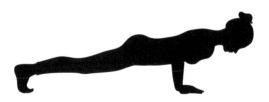

COBRA POSE

Bhujangasana

This pose is a wonderful stretch to open up your chest and stretch all across the front of your body. It stimulates your digestive organs, increases movement in your spine and strengthens your arms.

Step by step

1. Lie flat, with your forehead resting onto the mat, the tops of the feet flat to the mat and your feet together.

2. Place your hands underneath your shoulders, palms flat to the mat, fingers pointing forwards. Roll your chest up and away from the mat and feel your body lengthening from the base of your belly to your chest. Engage your thigh muscles and feel your knees lifting.

3. Start to press your pubic bone down and inhale as you lift your chest higher. Keep the tops of your feet pressing down and press your palms down as you straighten your arms, curling your spine up and raising your chest. Feel the arching movement in your back from the base of the spine to the middle of your back. Plant the heels of your hands into the mat so you feel almost like you are pulling your chest forwards.

4. Soften your shoulders, pulling them down your back, opening across the chest. Tuck your chin in towards your throat, keeping the neck long.

5. Hold for five deep breaths, expanding your chest and lengthening your spine with each breath. Exhale as you slowly lower all the way down to the mat.

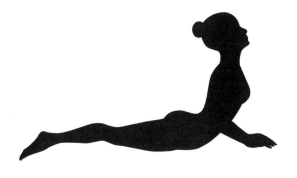

SUN SALUTATION A

Surya Namaskar A

Start in Mountain Pose (see page 40)

1. Inhale – Extended Mountain Pose: Mountain Pose
   with arms lifted above head

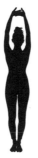

2. Exhale – Deep Forward Fold (see page 43)

3. Inhale – Half Forward Fold

4. Exhale – Walk, step or jump into a plank position and lower to Four-Limbed Staff Pose (see page 52). A lighter option is to lower the knees to the mat first then lower the chest.

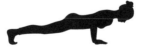

5. Inhale – Upward-Facing Dog (see page 49)

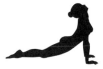

A lighter option is to take Cobra Pose (see page 54).

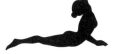

6. Exhale – Downward-Facing Dog (see page 46) Hold for three to five full and deep breaths.

7. Inhale – Walk, step or jump your feet between your hands – Half Forward Fold.

8. Exhale – Deep Forward Fold (see page 43)

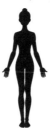

9. Inhale – Extended Mountain Pose

10. Exhale – Mountain Pose (see page 40)

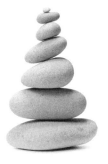

STANDING POSES

Now that you are fully warmed up the following postures can be attempted. It's imperative to read through the step-by-step instructions to make sure you are clear about each one. Don't forget to make sure you listen to your body and respond accordingly by, for example, not over-stretching and making small adjustments to your alignment to avoid injury.

A good rule of thumb is to take a mixture of standing, seated and lying postures for each practice, working through them in that order. However, if you want a more dynamic practice you can add more standing and balancing postures, or for a more restorative practice work with more seated and lying postures. Make your practice what your body and mind needs.

CHAIR POSE

Utkatasana

Chair Pose works both your legs and arms, strengthening and toning your muscles in these areas, as well as stimulating your chest and diaphragm. It can be a test of your willpower as long breaths can be difficult to complete, but try to set yourself a target of five long breaths.

Step by step

1. Come to the top of your mat in Mountain Pose (see page 40). Take your feet hip distance apart, inhale as you lift your arms above your head, exhale as you fold forwards. Bend your knees and bring your chest towards your thighs, placing your hands on the mat above your toes.

2. Bend your knees a little deeper, bringing your thighs parallel to the mat, with your knees only slightly ahead of your ankles and pointing out over your toes, avoiding your knees knocking together. Plant your feet into the mat, as you do in Mountain Pose, and inhale as you lift your arms and your chest away from your thighs.

3. Keep lifting your chest as you extend through your fingers and arms, reaching towards the sky, and draw your shoulders down to open your chest.

4. Tuck your tailbone in, engaging your core as your navel draws back to your spine. Feel your back flattening out and keep your gaze forwards.

5. Hold this pose for five deep breaths. To release, inhale as you lift your arms, straighten your legs and exhale to bring your arms down back into Mountain Pose.

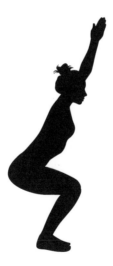

WARRIOR I POSE

Virabhadrasana I

As the name would suggest this is a strengthening and invigorating pose. The pose helps to increase focus and grounding, lifts and opens your chest, and gently tones your core and lower half of the body.

Step by step

1. Start in Mountain Pose (see page 40), step your left foot back so that your feet are wide apart. Ensure your right foot is pointing forwards, and your left foot is turned in about 45 degrees so that the heel is flat to the mat and the arch of your left foot is in line with the heel of your right foot.

2. Square your shoulders and hips to the front of your mat by drawing your left hip slightly forwards. Bend your right knee to 90 degrees, stacking your knee above your ankle, ensuring your knee does not pass your ankle or roll in or out.

3. Inhale as you lift your arms above your head and join your palms together. Draw your shoulders down from your ears, expanding across your chest. Take your gaze up towards your thumbs.

4. Ensure you spread your weight across both feet, grounding your left heel into the mat. Drop your

tailbone towards the floor, opening across the hips and lengthening your lower back.

5. Hold the pose for five deep breaths. Straighten your right leg and exhale as you take your hands down to heart centre. Step the left foot forwards to Mountain Pose. Repeat on the other side.

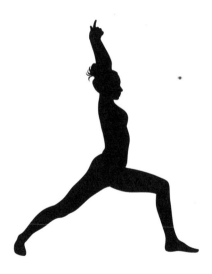

WARRIOR II POSE
Virabhadrasana II

Like Warrior I, this pose ignites your inner strength and tones your legs, as it relies on the power of your lower half to keep you standing strong while awakening your inner warrior.

Step by step

1. Stand in Mountain Pose (see page 40) at the top of your mat. Step your left foot back, taking your feet wide apart. Turn your left foot to 90 degrees, taking the arch of your left foot in line with the heel of your right foot.

2. Square your hips and shoulders forwards to the long edge of your mat, keeping your shoulders directly above your hips and your torso upright and facing forwards.

3. Raise your arms to shoulder level with your palms facing down, extend through the fingers and lower your shoulders from your ears, softening your upper back.

4. Turn your head to the right, taking your gaze out over the middle finger of your right hand. Bend your right knee so it is stacked above your ankle, ensuring the knee does not extend beyond the ankle and is not rolling inwards. You should feel a stretch to your inner thigh here.

5. Tuck your tailbone under, engaging your core. Lift and lengthen your spine, reaching the crown of your head to the sky. Ground your left foot into the mat, pressing into the outer edge of the foot and continue to extend through the fingers as you engage your inner warrior.

6. Take five deep breaths. Inhale as you straighten your right leg and take your gaze back to the front. Turn your right foot in and your left foot out, repeat on the other side.

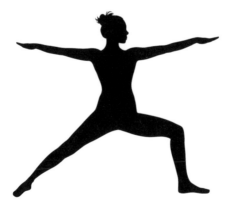

WARRIOR III POSE

Virabhadrasana III

As is the case with all balance postures,
not only does Warrior III strengthen
your legs and abdomen, it increases
focus and calms your mind.

Step by step

1. Start in Warrior I (see page 66) with your right leg forwards, pick up your left heel bringing yourself to the ball of your foot. Start to extend through your fingers, lifting your spine upwards. Exhale as you fold forwards, lowering your torso towards your right thigh, bringing your back and arms parallel with the floor. Lower your gaze and tuck your chin under, bringing your neck in line with your spine.

2. Ground your right foot into the floor, pushing through the big toe, ball and heel of your foot. Inhale as you slowly lift your left foot away from the floor, extending the left leg fully behind you. Keep your arms extended in front of you, palms together, fingers extended.

3. Draw your left hip towards the floor, keeping both hips parallel with the floor. Turn the toes of your lifted leg down towards the mat and press into your heel to lengthen through the back of your left leg.

4. Take your gaze ahead of your extended fingers. Keep your abdominal muscles engaged to support your centre of balance and take five deep breaths. To release, exhale as you slowly lower your left foot to the floor next to your right foot. Release your arms towards the floor and slowly roll up through the spine.

5. Step back into Warrior I with your left foot forwards and repeat on the other side.

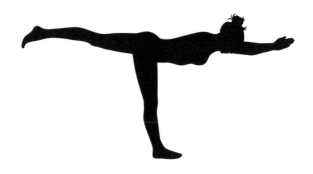

TRIANGLE POSE

Trikonasana

Triangle Pose is a wonderfully awakening, energising pose. It opens up your hips and chest, allowing for deep breathing and strengthening of your legs and torso.

Step by step

1. Stand in Mountain Pose (see page 40) at the top of your mat. Step your left foot back, taking your feet wide apart, and turn your left foot to 90 degrees, taking the arch of your left foot in line with the heel of your right foot.

2. Square your hips and shoulders forwards to the long edge of your mat, keeping your shoulders directly

above your hips and your trunk upright and facing forwards. Lengthen your spine as you draw your crown upwards.

3. Raise your arms to shoulder level with your palms facing down, extend your stretch through the fingers and lower your shoulders from your ears, softening your upper back.

4. Inhale and extend your upper body to the right, reaching your fingertips out over your toes, keeping your spine long. As you exhale, fold down over your right leg taking your right hand as low down your leg as you can. You can either hold onto your leg or if you have good balance keep your palm open with your fingers extending towards the floor. Alternatively, you may be able to take your palm all the way down to the floor to place it on the outside of your foot.

5. Extend through your left arm and with your palm facing forwards reach your fingertips towards the sky. Keep your arms in a straight line, in line with your

shoulders. Turn your gaze up towards your left palm.

6. Revolve your navel upwards. Open across your chest as you draw your left shoulder back and shift your hips forwards, taking your shoulder and hip in line with each other. Feel the lengthening across the left side of your torso.

7. Take five deep breaths. Inhale as you lift your upper body and take your gaze back to the front. Turn your right foot in and your left foot out. Repeat on the other side.

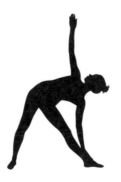

STANDING SIDE STRETCH POSE

Parsvakonasana

Side stretch poses open out areas of your body not used on a regular basis, thus working the inner and outer edges of both your extended arm and leg, and toning your thigh muscle.

Step by step

1. Stand in Mountain Pose (see page 40) at the top of your mat. Step your left foot back, taking your feet wide apart, and turn your left foot to 90 degrees, taking the arch of your left foot in line with the heel of your right foot.

2. Square your hips and shoulders forwards to the long edge of your mat, keeping your shoulders directly above your hips and your trunk upright and facing forwards. Lengthen your spine as you draw your crown upwards.

3. Raise your arms to shoulder level with your palms facing down, extend out through your fingers and lower your shoulders away from your ears, softening your upper back.

4. Inhale as you bend your knee, ensuring your knee is stacked above your ankle and not in front of the ankle. Exhale as you bend to the side, taking

the right ribs towards the right thigh; hug the ribs towards the thigh as you bring the palm of your hand to the floor on the outer side of your right foot. Alternatively you can rest your right forearm on your thigh, just above your knee.

5. Press your right leg back towards your arm, opening out the inner thigh, and revolve your trunk towards the sky.

6. Extend your left arm over your head, with your palm facing down and your fingertips extended to the side. Draw your left shoulder up and back to further open your chest and keep your trunk revolving towards the sky. Take your gaze up towards your left palm.

7. Ground your left foot into the mat, pressing into the outer edge of the foot, and continue to extend through your fingers, feeling the opening in your side right from your fingertips to your left heel.

8. Take five deep breaths. Inhale as you lift your upper body, straighten your right leg, and turn your right foot in and your left foot out. Repeat on the other side.

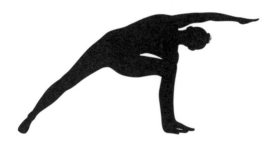

WIDE-LEGGED FORWARD FOLD POSE

Prasarita Padottanasana

Wide leg folds are wonderfully opening and satisfying stretches. This overall stretch elongates your hamstrings and spine, and encourages deeper breathing as your chest expands.

Step by step

1. Stand in Mountain Pose (see page 40) at the top of your mat. Step your left foot back, taking your feet wide apart, and turn both feet in slightly. Ground both feet into the mat, connecting to the mat with your toes, heels and the balls of both feet, similar to the grounding in Mountain Pose.

2. Square your hips and shoulders forwards to the long edge of your mat, keeping your shoulders directly above your hips and your trunk upright and facing forwards. Lengthen your spine as you draw your crown upwards.

3. Take your hands to your hips, inhale as you tuck your tailbone under, lengthen through your spine and open your chest. Exhale as you fold from the waist, tipping your tailbone back and keeping your spine long as you reach the crown of your head towards the ground.

4. Bring your hands to your mat, shoulder width apart and in line with your feet. Draw your shoulders back from your ears, lengthening the neck and spine.

5. Press into the outer edges of both feet as you draw your tailbone upwards. Draw your weight into the balls of your feet, stacking your hips, knees and ankles above each other. Feel the opening in the backs of your legs, extending your hamstrings.

6. Take five deep breaths. Inhale as you lift your upper body and step back to the top of your mat.

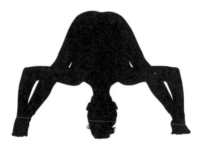

TREE POSE

Vrksasana

Tree Pose helps you to feel grounded and
strong as your feet and legs support you
like tree roots growing into the ground,
and your upper body lifts and lengthens
as your tree grows. As a balance posture
it is wonderful for calming your mind.

Step by step

1. Come to the top of your mat in Mountain Pose (see page 40). Take a moment to focus on your feet and their connection with your mat. Start to transfer your weight to your right foot, keeping it strong and grounded as you lift your left heel.

2. Bend your left knee and slowly turn it out to the side, opening your left hip. Place the heel of your left foot against your right leg as close to your upper inner thigh as possible. If you struggle to bring the foot to your upper thigh you can rest the sole of your foot onto the inside of your lower leg or onto your ankle with your big toe resting on the mat, however be sure to avoid resting your foot onto your knee.

3. Draw your left knee out further, opening across the hip, and gently draw your lower abdomen towards your spine, lengthening through your spine as you draw the crown of your head up. Ensure the sole of your foot is fully connected with your leg.

4. Bring the palms of your hands together at your heart centre, inhale as you slowly lift the arms, bringing your joined palms just above your head.

5. Keep your gaze forwards and ensure your breath is still long and steady – do not be tempted to hold your breath!

6. After five deep breaths slowly bring your joined palms back to your heart centre. Turn your left knee in to point forwards, point your left toes to the floor and slowly slide your left foot down to the mat. Repeat on the other side.

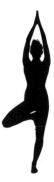

REMEMBER IT DOESN'T
MATTER HOW DEEP INTO A
POSTURE YOU GO – WHAT
MATTERS IS WHO YOU ARE
WHEN YOU GET THERE.

MAX STROM

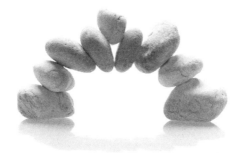

SEATED POSES

Over the next few pages you will find a
series of seated fold poses, which are
wonderful for calming the body and mind.
As the body folds in on itself you can
reconnect inwards, and open your chest to
stimulate deeper and slower breathing.

DEEP SEATED FORWARD FOLD POSE

Paschimottanasana

This pose offers an intense stretch to your back, gentle toning of your abdominal organs and opening to the backs of your legs.

Step by step

1. Start seated on your mat with your legs extended in front of you, toes pointing up, feet connected at the inner edges. Extend through your heels, activating the backs of your legs, pushing your calves and the backs of your knees towards the mat. Place your hands either side of your hips on the floor.

2. Tilt your weight slightly forwards, bringing yourself to the front of your sitting bones. Inhale as you lift your arms above your head, extending through your fingers and lengthening your spine upwards.

3. Exhale and engage your core, drawing your navel back towards your spine, as you fold your upper body over your legs. Keep your spine lengthening as you fold, extending your arms along your legs. Take hold of your big toes with your first two fingers or the outer edges of your feet with your hands. Alternatively you can take hold around your shins or ankles.

4. Avoid rounding your back. Draw your shoulders back from your ears, lengthen your spine and push your chest forwards. The forward fold motion should come from the base of your spine, not the middle of your back.

5. If you can reach your feet comfortably bend the elbows and fold deeper into the pose. Keep your neck in line with your spine by not dropping your head towards

your legs. Draw your shoulders back from your ears to lengthen through your neck and spine further.

6. Once you reach your maximum extensions, hold for five deep breaths, extending with each exhale and keep the backs of your legs in contact with the mat.

7. To release, inhale as you slowly roll up through your spine, lifting your arms above your head, and exhale to lower your arms back to your sides.

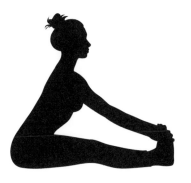

HEAD-TO-KNEE POSE

Janu Sirsasana

This pose tones your abdominal organs and opens your hips and the backs of your legs, allowing tension to release.

Step by step

1. Start seated on your mat with your legs extended in front of you, toes pointing up, feet connected at the inner edges. Extend through your heels, activating the backs of your legs. Draw your right knee up and turn it out to the side, bringing the sole of your foot to the inside of your left thigh.

2. Tilt your weight slightly forwards, bringing yourself to the front of your sitting bones. Inhale as you lift your arms above your head, extending through your fingers and lengthening your spine upwards. Slightly rotate your torso to line up with your left leg.

3. Exhale and engage your core, drawing your navel back towards your spine as you fold forwards. Keep your spine lengthening as you fold, extending your arms along your legs. Take hold around your foot, alternatively you can take hold around the shin or ankle.

4. Avoid rounding your back. Draw your shoulders back from your ears, lengthen your spine and push your chest forwards.

5. If you can reach your foot comfortably, bend your elbows and fold deeper into the pose. Draw your shoulders back from your ears to lengthen through your neck and spine further. Keep drawing the right knee back and down, opening out the hip as you breathe into the pose.

6. Once you reach your maximum extensions, hold for five deep breaths. To release, inhale as you slowly roll up through your spine, lifting your arms above your head, and exhale to lower your arms back to your sides. Use your hand to slowly draw your right knee up and then lower your leg down. Repeat on the other side.

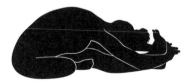

SAGE FORWARD BEND A POSE

Marichyasana A

This is a great pose for lengthening your hamstrings, opening your hips and stimulating both your abdominal and pelvic region.

Step by step

1. Start seated on your mat with your legs extended in front of you, toes pointing up. Bend your right knee up, bringing the sole of your foot flat to the mat next to your left thigh with roughly a fist-sized distance between the thigh and foot. Ensure your toes are pointing forwards and bring your heel close to your sitting bones.

2. Inhale as you lift your arms above your head, extending your fingers upwards. Tilt your body forwards, rolling to the front of your sitting bones. Exhale as you fold, taking your right arm to the inside of your right leg, and reach your arm forwards until you bring your armpit against your right shin.

3. Rotate your right arm so your palm is facing outwards and your thumb turns down towards the floor. Bend your elbow bringing your hand back and wrapping your arm around your bent leg.

4. Reach your left arm forwards, folding a little deeper towards your left leg. Then rotate your left arm, turning your palm to face outwards and take your arms back behind you to meet your right hand behind your back. Take hold of your left wrist with your right hand.

5. Alternatively if you struggle to meet your hands together you can use a yoga strap, placing the strap behind you before you begin and then holding onto the strap with each hand as you reach your hands behind the back.

6. Exhale as you lengthen forwards over the left leg, drawing your chest forwards and down and reaching the crown of your head towards your toes. Keep your left leg engaged, toes pointing up, with the back of your leg pressing into the floor.

7. Keep the sole of your right foot planted into the floor and your arms extending out behind you, and hold for five deep breaths.

8. To come out of this pose, release your hands from behind your back and exhale as you roll up. Take your right leg down and repeat on the other side.

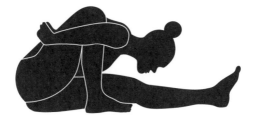

SEATED ANGLE FOLD POSE

Upavistha Konasana

This lovely opening pose provides a deep stretch to your inner thighs, legs and hips, as well as gently toning your abdomen and lower back.

Step by step

1. Start seated on your mat with your legs extended in front of you. Spread your legs wide apart, and push through your heels to straighten and activate the backs of your legs, turning your toes up and pushing the backs of your knees towards the mat. Place your hands either side of your hips on the floor. Ensure you keep your toes and knees pointing up and not rolling in or out throughout this pose.

2. Tilt your weight slightly forwards, lifting and opening your chest and slightly curving your lower back inwards. Then take a deep inhale.

3. Exhale as you lean forwards, engaging your core and drawing your navel back towards your spine. Take hold of your big toes with the first two fingers of each hand or hold around your legs or ankles. Try to notice both your back and spine lengthening forwards as well as your abdomen and chest, lengthening and opening both sides of your torso.

4. Bend your elbows as you fold deeper into the pose, bringing your forehead towards the mat between your feet. Draw your shoulders back from your ears to lengthen through your neck and spine further.

5. Once you reach your maximum extensions, hold for five deep breaths. Keep your breath slow and steady, allowing your body to come deeper into the pose with each exhale.

6. To release, inhale as you slowly roll up, walking your hands up your legs. Use your hands underneath your knees to gently bring your legs back together.

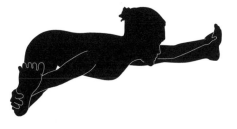

HAPPINESS IS WHEN WHAT YOU THINK, WHAT YOU SAY AND WHAT YOU DO ARE IN HARMONY.

MAHATMA GANDHI

BOAT POSE

Navasana

Boat Pose is deceptively challenging,
but one of the best poses for toning and
strengthening your abdomen, as well
as strengthening your lower back.

Step by step

1. Start seated on your mat with your knees bent, the soles of your feet flat to the mat and your hands either side of your hips on the floor. Lean back slightly, rolling to the outer edges of your sitting bones.

2. Start to lift your feet away from the mat, keeping your knees and feet in line with each other; continue to lift your feet, bending into your knees to bring your shins parallel to the floor.

3. Extend your arms out in front of you alongside your legs. Turn your palms in towards your legs and keep extending through your fingertips. Start to lift your chest, draw your shoulders back and your chest forwards.

4. Hold here, or to practise Full Boat Pose slowly start to straighten the legs upwards to their full extension. You'll need to keep working your abdominal muscles to ensure the chest is still drawing forwards and upwards to avoid rounding into the back and keeping the legs fully extended.

5. Hold for five deep breaths. To release, exhale as you slowly bend your knees and lower your toes towards the floor.

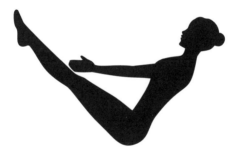

BRIDGE POSE

Setu Bandhasana

This back bend opens your chest and hips, and
strengthens your spine and the front of your
legs, and can aid some lower back problems.
It also helps to relieve stress and tension.

Step by step

1. Start by lying on your mat, arms to your sides, palms facing down. Bend your knees, placing the soles of your feet on the mat about hip distance apart. Take your feet back towards your sitting bones, keeping your toes pointing forwards.

2. Engage your abdominals and tilt your pelvis away from the mat, inhale as you lift your buttocks off the mat and push your hips upwards. Keep lifting your body away from the mat, planting the soles of your feet strongly into the ground.

3. Clasp your hands together underneath your body, extending your arms towards your feet. Keep lifting your hips higher as you roll onto the tops of your shoulders. Your little fingers should be flat on the mat with your knuckles extending towards your heels.

4. Ensure your knees stay in line with your hips and don't let your knees point out to the sides. Tuck your

chin under, keep your neck long and take your gaze towards your navel. Do not move your head or your neck while in this pose.

5. Hold for five deep breaths and keep drawing your hips upwards. To release, unclasp your hands, taking your arms back to your sides, and exhale as you slowly roll your spine back into the mat. Rest for a couple of breaths on the mat before moving your body.

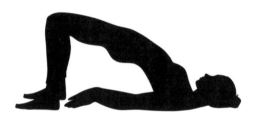

A TRULY FLEXIBLE BACK MAKES FOR A LONG LIFE.

CHINESE PROVERB

HAPPY BABY POSE
Ananda Balasana

Happy Baby Pose is great for opening your hips, and releasing tension and tightness from your hips and inner legs. It also lengthens your spine and gently stretches your whole back.

Step by step

1. Start by lying on your mat, arms to your sides, palms facing down. Bend your knees up into your chest, take your arms between your knees and take hold of the outside of your feet, alternatively you can hook your big toes with the first two fingers of each hand.

2. Draw your knees closer to your chest as you widen them apart, bringing your knees out towards your armpits. Take your feet shoulder width apart with the soles of your feet facing upwards, bringing your ankles in line with your knees.

3. Inhale as you pull your feet down, drawing your knees closer to your armpits. Exhale as you draw your shoulders and your tailbone towards the mat, tuck your chin under towards your chest and feel the lengthening of your neck and spine on the mat.

4. Hold for five deep breaths. Release your feet, bringing your knees together, hug your knees into your chest, exhale and lower your feet to the mat.

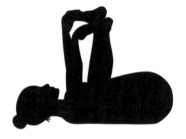

REVOLVED ABDOMEN POSE

Jathara Parivartanasana

This spinal twist gently squeezes your abdomen, toning it and releasing stored toxins. It is wonderful for relieving lower back pain and great for closing your practice before finishing in Corpse Pose (see page 19).

Step by step

1. Start lying flat on your mat, take your arms out to your sides at shoulder level, arms flat to the mat, palms facing down. Tuck your chin in towards your chest, lengthening the back of your neck and relax your shoulders.

2. Bring your knees into your chest, inhale and expand your chest then exhale as you lower your knees to your right side. Allow your feet to come to the floor and keep both shoulders flat to the mat. Keep your knees together then draw them up towards your chest, taking your knees in line with your hips.

3. Turn your head to the left and hold for several deep breaths. With each breath feel your spine lengthening and allow your body to revolve further, but keep your shoulders flat to the mat.

4. Slowly turn your head back to centre and inhale as you lift your knees back to your chest. Exhale as you lower your legs to the left and repeat on the left side.

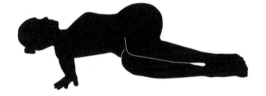

RECLINED BOUND ANGLE POSE

Supta Baddha Konasana

This pose opens your hips and inner thighs, helps to relieve digestive and reproductive disorders by increasing the blood supply to your pelvic area and opens your chest to promote deeper breathing.

Step by step

1. Start by lying flat on your mat, arms by your sides, palms facing up. Tuck your chin in towards your chest, lengthening the back of your neck.

2. Bend your knees up, bringing the soles of your feet flat to the mat. Open your knees allowing each to fall towards the mat, bringing the soles of your feet together. Ensure your neck is still in line with your spine and your shoulders are relaxed towards the mat.

3. See if you can bring your heels closer to your body, keeping your soles connected. Relax your hip sockets, allowing an opening on your inner thighs and letting gravity gently take control.

4. Soften your belly, allowing your chest and belly to gently rise and fall with your breath. Close your eyes, bring your attention inwards and allow your breath to deepen.

5. Stay here for several deep breaths, feeling your thighs and hips open a little more with each breath, releasing tension and tightness from the body.

6. Release slowly by bringing your knees together and hugging them to your chest.

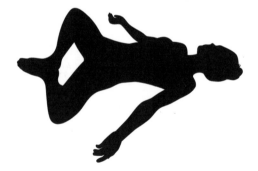

WHEN YOU FIND PEACE
WITHIN YOURSELF, YOU
BECOME THE KIND OF
PERSON WHO CAN LIVE AT
PEACE WITH OTHERS.

PEACE PILGRIM

CONCLUSION

I hope you have enjoyed *The Little Book of Yoga*
and are looking forward to starting your journey.

Namaste – the divine light within me
recognises the divine light within you.

ABOUT THE AUTHOR

I first started practicing yoga in my twenties when looking for something to improve my stress and anxiety related health issues. Nervous to go to class on my own and knowing all the stigmas attached to yoga I started practicing at home using online videos, it was a great way to start my yoga journey however I knew I wanted more. I had fallen in love with the practice and wanted to improve and deepen my yoga journey. My journey then took me to India to learn the traditional teachings of yoga and allow me to share the magic.

With this Little Book I hope to encourage some of you to start your yoga journey and enjoy all the benefits of this wonderful practice.

Index

Image credits